RENAL

Kidney Diet Cookbook for Newly Diagnosed Patients: The Complete Guide to Kidney Disease Management and Avoiding Dialysis

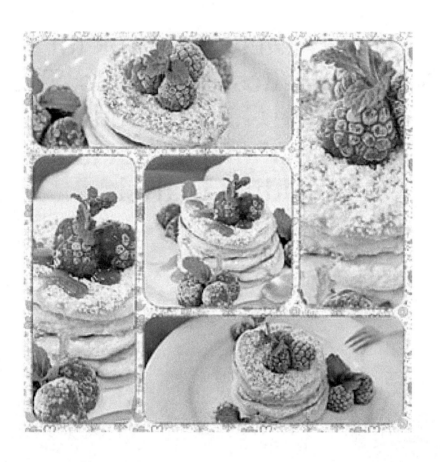

The information in the following pages is broadly considered a truthful and accurate account of facts and as such, any inattention, use, or misuse of the information in question by the reader will render any resulting actions solely under their purview. There are no scenarios in which the publisher or the original author of this work can be in any fashion deemed liable for any hardship or damages that may befall them after undertaking information described herein.

Additionally, the information in the following pages is intended only for informational purposes and should thus be thought of as universal. As befitting its nature, it is presented without assurance regarding its prolonged validity or interim quality. Trademarks that are mentioned are done without written consent and can in no way be considered an endorsement from the trademark holder.

TABLE OF CONTENTS

BREAKFAST

American Blueberry Pancakes

Preparation time: 5 minutes

Cooking time: 10 minutes

Servings: 6

Ingredients

- 1 ½ cups of all-purpose flour, sifted
- 1 cup of buttermilk
- 3 tablespoons of sugar
- 2 tablespoons of unsalted butter, melted
- 2 teaspoon of baking powder
- 2 eggs, beaten
- 1 cup of canned blueberries, rinsed

Directions

1. Combine the baking powder, flour and sugar in a bowl.

2. Make a hole in the center and slowly add the rest of the ingredients.

3. Begin to stir gently from the sides to the center with a spatula, until you get a smooth and creamy batter.

4. With cooking spray, spray the pan and place over medium heat.

5. Take one measuring cup and fill 1/3rd of its capacity with the batter to make each pancake.

6. Use a spoon to pour the pancake batter and let cook until golden brown. Flip once to cook the other side.

7. Serve warm with optional agave syrup.

Nutrition: calories: 251.69 kcal carbohydrate: 41.68 g protein: 7.2 g sodium: 186.68 mg potassium: 142.87 mg phosphorus: 255.39 mg dietary fiber: 1.9 g fat: 6.47 g

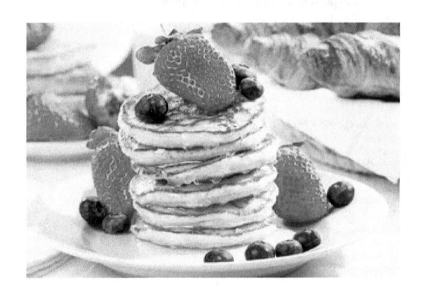

Raspberry Peach Breakfast Smoothie

Preparation time: 5 minutes

Cooking time: 1 minute

Servings: 2

Ingredients

- 1/3 cup of raspberries, (it can be frozen)
- 1/2 peach, skin and pit removed
- 1 tablespoon of honey
- 1 cup of coconut water

Directions

1. Mix all ingredients together and blend it until smooth.

2. Pour and serve chilled in a tall glass or mason jar.

Nutrition: calories: 86.3 kcal carbohydrate: 20.6 g protein: 1.4 g sodium: 3 mg potassium: 109 mg phosphorus: 36.08 mg dietary fiber: 2.6 g fat: 0.31 g

Fast Microwave Egg Scramble

Preparation time: 5 minutes

Cooking time: 1-2 minutes

Servings: 1

Ingredients

- 1 large egg
- 2 large egg whites
- 2 tablespoons of milk
- Kosher pepper, ground

Directions

1. Spray a coffee cup with a bit of cooking spray.

2. Whisk all the ingredients together and place into the coffee cup.

3. Place the cup with the eggs into the microwave and set to cook for approx. 45 seconds. Take out and stir.

4. Cook it for another 30 seconds after returning it to the microwave.

5. Serve.

Nutrition: calories: 128.6 kcal carbohydrate: 2.47 g protein: 12.96 g sodium: 286.36 mg potassium: 185.28 mg phosphorus: 122.22 mg dietary fiber: 0 g fat: 5.96 g

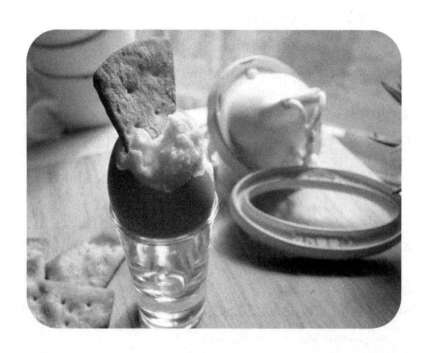

Mango Lassi Smoothie

Preparation time: 5 minutes

Cooking time: 0 minute

Servings: 2

Ingredients

- ½ cup of plain yogurt
- ½ cup of plain water
- ½ cup of sliced mango
- 1 tablespoon of sugar
- ¼ teaspoon of cardamom
- ¼ teaspoon cinnamon
- ¼ cup lime juice

Directions

1. Pulse all the above ingredients in a blender until smooth (around 1 minute).

2. Pour into tall glasses or mason jars and serve chilled immediately.

Nutrition: calories: 89.02 kcal carbohydrate: 14.31 g protein: 2.54 g sodium: 30 mg potassium: 185.67 mg phosphorus: 67.88 mg dietary fiber: 0.77 g fat: 2.05 g

Breakfast Maple Sausage

Preparation time: 15 minutes

Cooking time: 8 minutes

Servings: 12

Ingredients

- 1 pound of pork, minced
- ½ pound lean turkey meat, ground
- ¼ teaspoon of nutmeg
- ½ teaspoon black pepper
- ¼ all spice
- 2 tablespoon of maple syrup
- 1 tablespoon of water

Directions

1. Combine all the ingredients in a bowl.

2. Cover and refrigerate for 3-4 hours.

3. Take the mixture and form into small flat patties with your hand (around 10-12 patties).

4. Lightly grease a medium skillet with oil and shallow fry the patties over medium to high heat, until brown (around 4-5 minutes on each side).

5. Serve hot.

Nutrition: calories: 53.85 kcal carbohydrate: 2.42 g protein: 8.5 g sodium: 30.96 mg potassium: 84.68 mg phosphorus: 83.49 mg dietary fiber: 0.03 g fat: 0.9 g

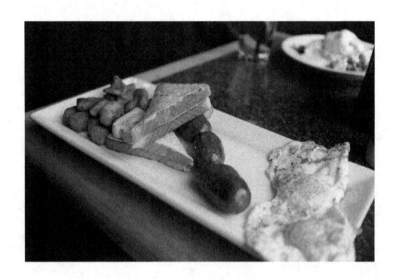

Summer Veggie Omelet

Preparation time: 5 minutes

Cooking time: 5 minutes

Servings: 2

Ingredients

- 4 large egg whites
- ¼ cup of sweet corn, frozen
- 1/3 cup of zucchini, grated
- 2 green onions, sliced
- 1 tablespoon of cream cheese
- Kosher pepper

Directions

1. Grease a medium pan with some cooking spray and add the onions, corn and grated zucchini.

2. Sauté for a couple of minutes until softened.

3. Beat the eggs together with the water, cream cheese, and pepper in a bowl.

4. Add the eggs into the veggie mixture in the pan, and let cook while moving the edges from inside to outside with a spatula, to allow raw egg to cook through the edges.

5. Turn the omelet with the aid of a dish (placed over the pan and flipped upside down and then back to the pan).

6. Let sit for another 1-2 minutes.

7. Fold in half and serve.

Nutrition: calories: 90 kcal carbohydrate: 15.97 g protein: 8.07 g sodium: 227 mg potassium: 244.24 mg phosphorus: 45.32 mg dietary fiber: 0.88 g fat: 2.44 g

Raspberry Overnight Porridge

Preparation time: overnight

Cooking time: 0 minute

Servings:12

Ingredients

- 1/3 cup of rolled oats
- ½ cup almond milk
- 1 tablespoon of honey
- 5-6 raspberries, fresh or canned and unsweetened
- 1/3 cup of rolled oats
- ½ cup almond milk
- 1 tablespoon of honey
- 5-6 raspberries, fresh or canned and unsweetened

Directions

1. Combine the oats, almond milk, and honey in a mason jar and place into the fridge for overnight.

2. Serve the next morning with the raspberries on top.

Nutrition: calories: 143.6 kcal carbohydrate: 34.62 g protein: 3.44 g sodium: 77.88 mg potassium: 153.25 mg phosphorus: 99.3 mg dietary fiber: 7.56 g fat: 3.91 g

Broccoli Rice Gratin (Italian Style)

Preparation Time: 30 minutes

Cooking Time: 47 minutes

Serving: 2

Ingredients:

- 125 g (10-minute rice
- salt
- 300 g broccoli florets
- salt
- from the mill: pepper
- 1 teaspoon dried Italian herb
- 1 teaspoon (noble sweet variety) paprika powder
- 125 g (8.5% fat) small mozzarella balls
- 2 tbsp pine nuts
- some basil leaves

Direction:

1. Following the directions on the packet, cook the rice with plenty of salted water. Meanwhile, clean the broccoli

florets and wash them, and cut them into smaller pieces. Add the broccoli to the rice about 5 minutes before cooking time ends, bring it all to a boil again, and simultaneously cook the broccoli.

2. Set the oven to 220 ° C. Brush baking dish (20 x 30 cm approx.) with oil. Drain in a colander with the rice and broccoli and drain. Use salt, pepper, Italian herbs, and paprika powder to season the bell pepper. Mix and dissolve in the baking dish with the broccoli rice mix.

3. Rinse and chop cherry bell pepper in half. Halve the balls of mozzarella as well. Combine the bell pepper and mozzarella, sprinkle with the pine nuts, and spread on the broccoli-rice mix. On the middle rack, bake the gratin in the oven for about 10 minutes. To serve, sprinkle with the basil leaves.

Nutrition: 320 calories 18g protein 45mg potassium 142mg sodium

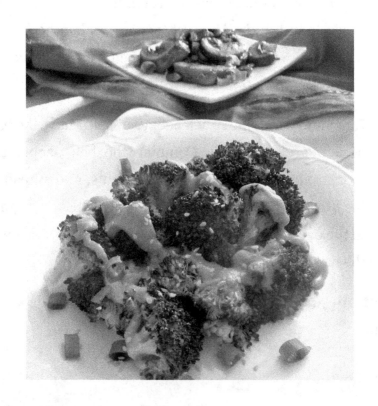

LUNCH

Crispy Lemon Chicken

Preparation Time: 10 minutes

Cooking Time: 10 minutes

Servings: 6

Ingredients:

- 1 lb. boneless and skinless chicken breast
- ½ cup of all-purpose flour
- 1 large egg
- ½ cup of lemon juice
- 2 tbsp. of water
- ¼ tsp salt
- ¼ tsp lemon pepper
- 1 tsp of mixed herb seasoning
- 2 tbsp. of olive oil
- A few lemon slices for garnishing
- 1 tbsp. of chopped parsley (for garnishing)
- 2 cups of cooked plain white rice

Directions:

1. Slice the chicken breast into thin and season with the herb, salt, and pepper.

2. In a small bowl, whisk together the egg with the water.

3. Keep the flour in a separate bowl.

4. Dip the chicken slices in the egg bath and then into the flour.

5. Heat your oil in a medium frying pan.

6. Shallow fry the chicken in the pan until golden brown.

7. Add the lemon juice and cook for another couple of minutes.

8. Taken the chicken out of the pan and transfer on a wide dish with absorbing paper to absorb any excess oil.

9. Garnish with some chopped parsley and lemon wedges on top.

10. Serve with rice.

Nutrition: Calories: 232 Carbohydrate: 24g Protein: 18g Fat: 8g Sodium: 100g Potassium: 234mg Phosphorus: 217mg

Mexican Steak Tacos

Preparation Time: 10 minutes

Cooking Time: 15 minutes

Servings: 8

Ingredients:

- 1 pound of flank or skirt steak
- ¼ cup of fresh cilantro, chopped
- ¼ cup white onion, chopped
- 3 limes, juiced
- 3 cloves of garlic, minced
- 2 tsp of garlic powder
- 2 tbsp. of olive oil
- ½ cup of Mexican or mozzarella cheese, grated
- 1 tsp of Mexican seasoning
- 8 medium-sized (6") corn flour tortillas

Directions:

1. Combine the juice from two limes, Mexican seasoning, and garlic powder in a dish or bowl and marinate the steak with it for at least half an hour in the fridge.

2. In a separate bowl, combine the chopped cilantro, garlic, onion, and juice from one lime to make your salsa. Cover and keep in the fridge.

3. Slice steak into thin strips and cook for approximately 3 minutes on each side.

4. Preheat your oven to 350F/180C.

5. Distribute evenly the steak strips in each tortilla. Top with a tablespoon of the grated cheese on top.

6. Wrap each taco in aluminum foil and bake in the oven for 7-8 minutes or until cheese is melted.

7. Serve warm with your cilantro salsa.

Nutrition: Calories: 230 Carbohydrate: 19.5 g Protein: 15 g Fat: 11 g Sodium: 486.75 g Potassium: 240 mg Phosphorus: 268 mg

Beer Pork Ribs

Preparation Time: 10 minutes

Cooking Time: 8 hours

Servings: 1

Ingredients:

- 2 pounds of pork ribs, cut into two units/racks
- 18 oz. of root beer
- 2 cloves of garlic, minced
- 2 tbsp. of onion powder
- 2 tbsp. of vegetable oil (optional)

Directions:

1. Wrap the pork ribs with vegetable oil and place one unit on the bottom of your slow cooker with half of the minced garlic and the onion powder.

2. Place the other rack on top with the rest of the garlic and onion powder.

3. Pour over the root beer and cover the lid.

4. Let simmer for 8 hours on low heat.

5. Take off and finish optionally in a grilling pan for a nice sear.

Nutrition: Calories: 301 Carbohydrate: 36 g Protein: 21 g Fat: 18 g Sodium: 729 mg Potassium: 200 mg Phosphorus: 209 mg

Mexican Chorizo Sausage

Preparation Time: 10 minutes

Cooking Time: 15 minutes

Servings: 1

Ingredients:

- 2 pounds of boneless pork but coarsely ground
- 3 tbsp. of red wine vinegar
- 2 tbsp. of smoked paprika
- ½ tsp of cinnamon
- ½ tsp of ground cloves
- ¼ tsp of coriander seeds
- ¼ tsp ground ginger
- 1 tsp of ground cumin
- 3 tbsp. of brandy

Directions:

1. In a large mixing bowl, combine the ground pork with the seasonings, brandy, and vinegar and mix with your hands well.

2. Place the mixture into a large Ziploc bag and leave in the fridge overnight.

3. Form into 15-16 patties of equal size.

4. Heat the oil in a large pan and fry the patties for 5-7 minutes on each side, or until the meat inside is no longer pink and there is a light brown crust on top.

5. Serve hot.

Nutrition: Calories: 134Carbohydrate: 0 g Protein: 10 g Fat: 7 g

Sodium: 40 mg Potassium: 138 mg Phosphorus: 128 mg

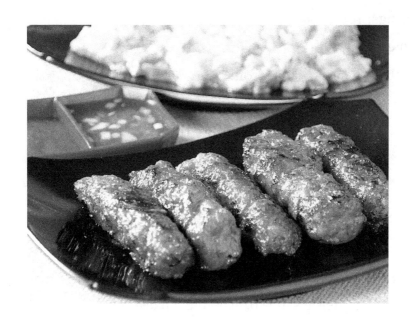

DINNER

Baked Macaroni & Cheese

Preparation Time: 10 minutes

Cooking Time: 40 – 45 minutes

Servings: 1

Ingredients:

- 3 cups of macaroni
- 2 cups of milk
- 2 tbsp of butter (unsalted)
- 2 tbsp of flour (all-purpose)
- 2 ½ cups of cheddar
- 2 tbsp of blanched almonds
- 1 tbsp of thyme
- 1 tbsp of olive oil
- 1 cheese sauce (quick make packets)

Directions:

1. Preheat the oven to 350 degrees-Fahrenheit.

2. Prepare a medium-sized pot on the stove and fill it up with water.

3. Add the macaroni to the pot with a tbsp of olive oil for 8-10 minutes. Stir until cooked.

4. In a measuring cup, measure your butter and flour and mix it. Place it in the microwave for 1 minute. Then stir in the milk, spices, and herbs—microwave for 2-3 minutes, or until the mixture is thick.

5. Drain the noodles and add to a casserole dish that has been sprayed with cooking spray, the sauce, and cheese. Mix it well, followed with more cheese on top.

6. Put and bake casserole dish into the oven for 15-20 minutes.

7. Serve with blanched almonds on top.

Nutrition: Calories: 314Fat: 14gCarbs: 34gProtein: 19g Sodium: 373mg Potassium: 120mgPhosphorus: 222mg

Korean Pear Salad

Preparation Time: 5 minutes

Cooking Time: 15 minutes

Servings: 2

Ingredients:

- 6 cups green lettuce
- 4 medium-sized pears (peeled, cored, and diced)
- ½ cup of sugar
- ½ cup of pecan nuts
- ½ cup of water
- 2 oz of blue cheese
- ½ cup of cranberries
- ½ cup of dressing

Directions:

1. Dissolve the water and sugar in a frying pan (non-stick).

2. Heat the mixture until it turns into a syrup, and then add the nuts immediately.

3. Place the syrup with the nuts on a piece of parchment paper and separate the nuts while the mixture is hot. Let it cool down.

4. Prepare lettuce in a salad bowl and add the pears, blue cheese, and cranberries to the salad.

5. Add the caramelized nuts to the salad and serve it with a dressing of choice on the side.

Nutrition: Calories: 112Fat: 9gCarbs: 5.5gProtein: 2gSodium: 130mg Potassium: 160mg Phosphorus: 71.7mg

Beef Enchiladas

Preparation Time: 10 minutes

Cooking Time: 30 minutes

Servings: 1

Ingredients:

- 1 pound of lean beef
- 12 whole-wheat tortillas
- 1 can of low-sodium enchilada sauce
- ½ cup of onion (diced)
- ½ tsp of black pepper
- 1 garlic clove
- 1 tbsp of olive oil
- 1 tsp of cumin

Directions:

1. Heat the oven to 375 degrees-Fahrenheit

2. In a medium-sized frying pan, cook the beef in olive oil until completely cooked.

3. Add the minced garlic, diced onion, cumin, and black pepper to the pan and mix everything in with the beef.

4. In a separate pan, cook the tortillas in olive oil and dip each cooked tortilla in the enchilada sauce.

5. Fill the tortilla with the meat mixture and roll it up.

6. Put the finished product in a slightly heated pan with cheese on top.

7. Bake the tortillas in the pan until crispy, golden brown, and the cheese is melted.

Nutrition: Calories: 177Fat: 6gCarbs: 15gProtein: 15gSodium: 501mg Potassium: 231mg Phosphorus: 98mg

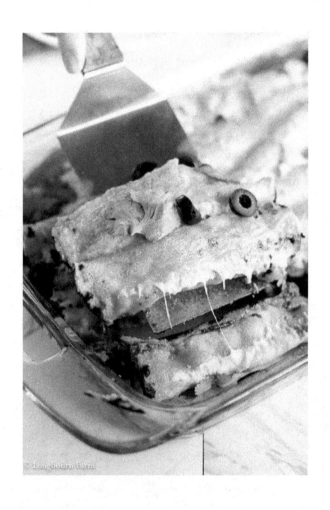

MAIN DISHES

Almond Scones

Preparation Time: 10 minutes

Cooking Time: 20 minutes

Servings: 6

Ingredients:

- 1 cup almonds
- 1 1/3 cups almond flour
- ¼ cup arrowroot flour
- 1 tablespoon coconut flour
- 1 teaspoon ground turmeric
- Salt, to taste
- Freshly ground black pepper, to taste
- 1 egg
- ¼ cup essential olive oil
- 3 tablespoons raw honey
- 1 teaspoon vanilla flavoring

Directions:

1. In a mixer, put almonds then pulse till chopped roughly
2. Move the chopped almonds in a big bowl.
3. Put flours and spices and mix well.

4. In another bowl, put the remaining ingredients and beat till well combined.
5. Put the flour mixture into the egg mixture then mix till well combined.
6. Arrange a plastic wrap over the cutting board.
7. Place the dough over the cutting board.
8. Using both of your hands, pat into 1-inch thick circle.
9. Cut the circle in 6 wedges.
10. Set the scones onto a cookie sheet in a single layer.
11. Bake for at least 15-20 minutes.

Nutrition: Calories: 304 Fat: 3gCarbohydrates: 22g Fiber: 6g Protein: 20g

Oven-Poached Eggs

Preparation Time: 2minutes

Cooking Time: 11minutes

Servings: 4

Ingredients:

- 6 eggs, at room temperature
- Water
- Ice bath
- 2 cups water, chilled
- 2 cups of ice cubes

Directions:

1. Set the oven to 350°F. Put 2 cups of water into a deep roasting tin, and place it into the lowest rack of the oven.

2. Place one egg into each cup of cupcake/muffin tins, along with one tablespoon of water.

3. Carefully place muffin tins into the middle rack of the oven.

4. Bake eggs for 45 minutes.

5. Turn off the heat immediately. Take off the muffin tins from the oven and set on a cake rack to cool before extracting eggs.

6. Pour ice bath ingredients into a large heat-resistant bowl.

7. Bring the eggs into an ice bath to stop the cooking process. After 10 minutes, drain eggs well. Use as needed.

Nutrition: Calories: 357 kcalProtein: 17.14 g Fat: 24.36 g Carbohydrates: 16.19 g

Cranberry and Raisins Granola

Preparation Time: 15 minutes

Cooking Time: 20 minutes

Servings: 4

Ingredients:

- 4 cups old-fashioned rolled oats
- 1/4 cup sesame seeds
- 1 cup dried cranberries
- 1 cup golden raisins
- 1/8 teaspoon nutmeg
- 2 tablespoons olive oil
- 1/2 cup almonds, slivered
- 2 tablespoons warm water
- 1 teaspoon vanilla extract
- 1 teaspoon cinnamon
- 1/4 teaspoon of salt
- 6 tablespoons maple syrup
- 1/3 cup of honey

Directions:

1. In a bowl, mix the sesame seeds, nutmeg, almonds, oats, salt, and cinnamon.
2. In another bowl, mix the oil, water, vanilla, honey, and syrup. Gradually pour the mixture into the oats mixture. Toss to combine. Spread the mixture into a

greased jelly-roll pan. Bake in the oven at 300°F for at least 55 minutes. Stir and break the clumps every 10 minutes.

3. Once you get it from the oven, stir the cranberries and raisins. Allow cooling. This will last for a week when stored in an airtight container and up to a month when stored in the fridge.

Nutrition: Calories: 698 kcal Protein: 21.34 g Fat: 20.99 g Carbohydrates: 148.59 g

SNACKS

Veggie Snack

Preparation Time: 5 minutes

Cooking Time: 10 minutes

Servings: 1

Ingredients:

- 1 large yellow pepper
- 5 carrots
- 5 stalks celery

Directions:

1. Clean the carrots and rinse under running water.

2. Rinse celery and yellow pepper. Remove seeds of pepper and chop the veggies into small sticks.

3. Put in a bowl and serve.

Nutrition: Calories: 189 Fat: 0.5 gCarbs: 44.3 g Protein: 5 g Sodium: 282 mg Potassium: 0mg Phosphorus: 0mg

Healthy Spiced Nuts

Preparation Time: 10 minutes

Cooking Time: 10 minutes

Servings: 4

Ingredients:

- 1 tbsp. extra virgin olive oil
- ¼ cup walnuts
- ¼ cup pecans
- ¼ cup almonds
- ½ tsp. sea salt
- ½ tsp. cumin
- ½ tsp. pepper
- 1 tsp. chili powder

Directions:

1. Put the skillet on medium heat and toast the nuts until lightly browned.

2. Prepare the spice mixture and add black pepper, cumin, chili, and salt.

3. Put extra virgin olive oil and sprinkle with spice mixture to the toasted nuts before serving.

Nutrition: Calories: 88 Fat: 8g Carbs: 4g Protein: 2.5gSodium: 51mg Potassium: 88mg Phosphorus: 6.3mg

Roasted Asparagus

Preparation Time: 5 minutes

Cooking Time: 10 minutes

Servings: 4

Ingredients:

- 1 tbsp. extra virgin olive oil
- 1-pound fresh asparagus
- 1 medium lemon, zested
- 1/2 tsp. freshly grated nutmeg
- 1/2 tsp. kosher salt
- ½ tsp. black pepper

Directions:

1. Preheat your oven to 500 degrees F.

2. Put asparagus on an aluminum foil and add extra virgin olive oil.

3. Prepare asparagus in a single layer and fold the edges of the foil.

4. Cook in the oven for 5 minutes. Continue roasting until browned.

5. Add the roasted asparagus with nutmeg, salt, zest, and pepper before serving.

Nutrition: Calories: 55Fat: 3.8 gCarbs: 4.7 gProtein: 2.5 g Sodium: 98mg Potassium: 172mg Phosphorus: 35mg

Low-Fat Mango Salsa

Preparation Time: 10 minutes

Cooking Time: 10 minutes

Servings: 4

Ingredients:

- 1 cup cucumber, chopped

- 2 cups mango, diced

- ½ cup cilantro, minced

- 2 tablespoons fresh lime juice

- 1 tablespoon scallions, minced

- ¼ teaspoon chipotle powder

- ¼ teaspoon sea salt

Directions

1. Mix the ingredients in a bowl and serve or refrigerate.

Nutrition: Calories: 155Fat: 0.6 g Carbs: 38.2 g Protein: 1.4 Sodium: 3.2 mg Potassium: 221mg Phosphorus: 27mg

Vinegar & Salt Kale

Preparation Time: 10 minutes

Cooking Time: 12 minutes

Servings: 2

Ingredients:

- 1 head kale, chopped
- 1 teaspoon extra virgin olive oil
- 1 tablespoon apple cider vinegar
- ½ teaspoon of sea salt

Directions:

2. Prepare kale in a bowl and put vinegar and extra virgin olive oil.

3. Sprinkle with salt and massage the ingredients with hands.

4. Spread the kale out onto two paper-lined baking sheets and bake at 375°F for about 12 minutes or until crispy.

5. Let cool for about 10 minutes before serving.

Nutrition: Calories: 152 Fat: 8.2 g Carbs: 15.2 g Protein: 4 g Sodium: 170mg Potassium: 304mg Phosphorus: 37mg

SOUP AND STEW

Thai Chicken Soup

Preparation Time: 10 minutes

Cooking Time: 30 minutes

Servings: 6

Ingredients:

- 4 chicken breasts, slice into 1/4-inch strips

- 1 tbsp. fresh basil, chopped

- 1 tsp ground ginger

- 1 oz. fresh lime juice

- 1 tbsp. coconut aminos

- 2 tbsp. chili garlic paste

- 1/4 cup fish sauce

- 28 oz. water

- 14 oz. chicken broth

- 14 oz. coconut almond milk

Directions:

1. Add coconut almond milk, basil, ginger, lime juice, coconut aminos, chili garlic paste, fish sauce, water, and broth into the stockpot. Stir well and bring to boil over medium-high heat.

2. Add chicken and stir well. Turn heat to medium-low and simmer for 30 minutes.

3. Stir well and serve.

Nutrition: Calories 357 Fat 23.4 g Carbohydrates 5.5 g Sugar 2.9 g Protein 31.7 g Cholesterol 87 mg Phosphorus: 110mg Potassium: 117mg Sodium: 75mg

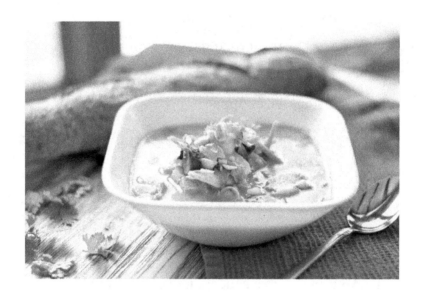

Tasty Pumpkin Soup

Preparation Time: 10 minutes

Cooking Time: 30 minutes

Servings: 6

Ingredients:

- 2 cups pumpkin puree
- 1 cup coconut cream
- 4 cups vegetable broth
- 1/2 tsp ground ginger
- 1 tsp curry powder
- 2 shallots, chopped
- 1/2 onion, chopped
- 4 tbsp. butter
- Pepper
- Salt

Directions:

1. Melt butter in a saucepan over medium heat.

2. Add shallots and onion and sauté until softened.

3. Add ginger and curry powder and stir well.

4. Add broth, pumpkin puree, and coconut cream and stir well. Simmer for 10 minutes.

5. Puree the soup using an immersion blender until smooth.

6. Season with pepper and salt.

7. Serve and enjoy.

Nutrition: Calories 229 Fat 18.4 g Carbohydrates 13 g Sugar 4.9 g Protein 5.6 g Cholesterol 20 mg Phosphorus: 120mg Potassium: 137mg Sodium: 95mg

Easy Zucchini Soup

Preparation Time: 10 minutes

Cooking Time: 25 minutes

Servings: 4

Ingredients:

- 5 zucchinis, sliced
- 8 oz. cream cheese, softened
- 5 cups vegetable stock
- Pepper
- Salt

Directions:

1. Add zucchini and stock into the stockpot and bring to boil over high heat.

2. Turn heat to medium and simmer for 20 minutes.

3. Add cream cheese and stir until cheese is melted.

4. Puree soup using an immersion blender until smooth.

5. Season with pepper and salt.

6. Serve and enjoy.

Nutrition: Calories 245 Fat 20.3 g Carbohydrates 10.9 g Sugar 5.2 g Protein 7.7 g Cholesterol 62 mg Phosphorus: 110mg Potassium: 117mg Sodium: 75mg

Quick Tomato Soup

Preparation Time: 10 minutes

Cooking Time: 5 minutes

Servings: 4

Ingredients:

- 28 oz. can tomato, diced

- 1 tbsp. balsamic vinegar

- 1 tbsp. dried basil

- 1 tbsp. dried oregano

- 1 tsp garlic, minced

- 2 tbsp. olive oil

- Pepper

- Salt

Directions:

1. Heat oil in a saucepan over medium heat.

2. Add basil, oregano, and garlic and saute for 30 seconds.

3. Add Red bell peppers, vinegar, pepper, and salt and simmer for 3 minutes.

4. Stir well and serve hot.

Nutrition: Calories 108 Fat 7.1 g Carbohydrates 11.2 g Sugar 6.8 g Protein 2 g Cholesterol 0 mg Phosphorus: 130mg Potassium: 127mg Sodium: 75mg

VEGETABLE

Thai Tofu Broth

Preparation time: 5 minutes

Cooking time: 15 minutes

Servings: 4 servings

Ingredients:

- 1 cup rice noodles
- ½ sliced onion
- 6 oz. drained, pressed and cubed tofu
- ¼ cup sliced scallions
- ½ cup water
- ½ cup chestnuts
- ½ cup rice almond milk
- 1 tbsp. lime juice
- 1 tbsp. coconut oil
- ½ finely sliced chili
- 1 cup snow peas

Directions:

1. Heat the oil in a wok on a high heat and then sauté the tofu until brown on each side.

2. Add the onion and sauté for 2-3 minutes.

3. Add the rice almond milk and water to the wok until bubbling.

4. Lower to medium heat and add the noodles, chili and water chestnuts.

5. Allow to simmer for 10-15 minutes and then add the sugar snap peas for 5 minutes.

6. Serve with a sprinkle of scallions.

Nutrition: Calories: 304 kcal; Total Fat: 13 g; Saturated Fat: 0 g; Cholesterol: 0 mg; Sodium: 36 mg; Total Carbs: 38 g; Fiber: 0 g; Sugar: 0 g; Protein: 9 g

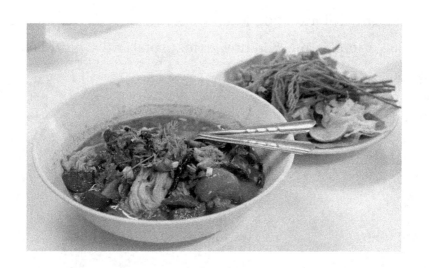

Delicious Vegetarian Lasagne

Preparation time: 10 minutes

Cooking time: 1 hour

Servings: 4 servings

Ingredients:

- 1 tsp. basil
- 1 tbsp. olive oil
- ½ sliced red pepper
- 3 lasagna sheets
- ½ diced red onion
- ¼ tsp. black pepper
- 1 cup rice almond milk
- 1 minced garlic clove
- 1 cup sliced eggplant
- ½ sliced zucchini
- ½ pack soft tofu
- 1 tsp. oregano

Directions:

1. Preheat oven to 325°F/Gas Mark 3.

2. Slice zucchini, eggplant and pepper into vertical strips.

3. Add the rice almond milk and tofu to a food processor and blitz until smooth. Set aside.

4. Heat the oil in a skillet over medium heat and add the onions and garlic for 3-4 minutes or until soft.

5. Sprinkle in the herbs and pepper and allow to stir through for 5-6 minutes until hot.

6. Into a lasagne or suitable oven dish, layer 1 lasagna sheet, then 1/3 the eggplant, followed by 1/3 zucchini, then 1/3 pepper before pouring over 1/3 of tofu white sauce.

7. Repeat for the next 2 layers, finishing with the white sauce.

8. Add to the oven for 40-50 minutes or until veg is soft and easily be sliced into servings.

Nutrition: Calories: 235 kcal; Total Fat: 9 g; Saturated Fat: 0 g; Cholesterol: 0 mg; Sodium: 35 mg; Total Carbs: 10 g; Fiber: 0 g; Sugar: 0 g; Protein: 5 g

Chili Tofu Noodles

Preparation time: 5 minutes

Cooking Time: 15 minutes

Servings: 4 servings

Ingredients:

- ½ diced red chili
- 2 cups rice noodles
- ½ juiced lime
- 6 oz. pressed and cubed silken firm tofu
- 1 tsp. grated fresh ginger
- 1 tbsp. coconut oil
- 1 cup green beans
- 1 minced garlic clove

Directions:

1. Steam the green beans for 10-12 minutes or according to package directions and drain.

2. Cook the noodles in a pot of boiling water for 10-15 minutes or according to package directions.

3. Meanwhile, heat a wok or skillet on a high heat and add coconut oil.

4. Now add the tofu, chili flakes, garlic and ginger and sauté for 5-10 minutes.

5. Drain the noodles and add to the wok along with the green beans and lime juice.

6. Toss to coat.

7. Serve hot!

Nutrition: Calories: 246 kcal; Total Fat: 12 g; Saturated Fat: 0 g; Cholesterol: 0 mg; Sodium: 25 mg; Total Carbs: 28 g; Fiber: 0 g; Sugar: 0 g; Protein: 10 g

SIDE DISHES

Cinnamon Apple Chips

Preparation Time: 5 minutes

Cooking Time: 2 to 3 hours

Servings: 4

Ingredients:

- 4 apples
- 1 teaspoon ground cinnamon

Directions:

1. Preheat the oven to 200°F. Line a baking sheet with parchment paper.
2. Core the apples and cut into 1/8-inch slices.
3. In a medium bowl, toss the apple slices with the cinnamon. Spread the apples in a single layer on the prepared baking sheet.
4. Cook for 2 to 3 hours, until the apples are dry. They will still be soft while hot, but will crisp once completely cooled.
5. Store in an airtight container for up to four days.
6. Cooking tip: If you don't have parchment paper, use cooking spray to prevent sticking.

Nutrition: Calories: 96; Total Fat: 0g; Saturated Fat: 0g; Cholesterol: 0mg; Carbohydrates: 26g; Fiber: 5g; Protein: 1g; Phosphorus: 0mg; Potassium: 198mg; Sodium: 2mg

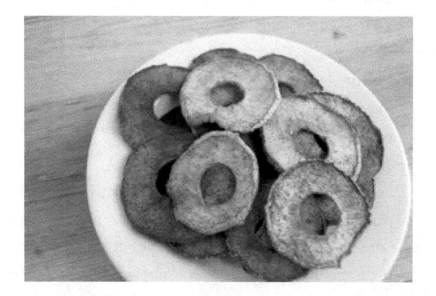

Roasted Red Pepper Hummus

Preparation Time: 10 minutes

Cooking Time: 10 minutes

Servings: 28

Ingredients:

- 1 red bell pepper
- 1 (15-ounce) can chickpeas, drained and rinsed
- Juice of 1 lemon
- 2 tablespoons tahini
- 2 garlic cloves
- 2 tablespoons extra-virgin olive oil

Directions:

1. Change an oven rack to the highest position. Heat the broiler to high.
2. Core the pepper and cut it into three or four large pieces. Arrange them on a baking sheet, skin-side up.
3. Broil the peppers for 5 to 10 minutes, until the skins are charred.
4. Cover with plastic wrap and let them steam for 10 to 15 minutes, until cool enough to handle.
5. Peel the skin off the peppers, and place the peppers in a blender.
6. Add the chickpeas, lemon juice, tahini, garlic, and olive oil.

7. Process until smooth, adding up to 1 tablespoon of water to adjust consistency as desired.

8. Substitution tip: This hummus can also be made without the red pepper if desired. To do this, simply follow Step 5. This will cut the potassium to 59mg per serving.

Nutrition: Total Fat: 6g; Saturated Fat: 1g; Cholesterol: 0mg; Carbohydrates: 10g; Fiber: 3g; Protein: 3g; Phosphorus: 58mg; Potassium: 91mg; Sodium: 72mg

SALAD

Hawaiian Chicken Salad

Preparation time: 5 minutes

Cooking time: 30 minutes

Servings: 4

Ingredients:

- 1 1/2 cups of chicken breast, cooked, chopped
- 1 cup pineapple chunks
- 1 1/4 cups lettuce iceberg, shredded
- 1/2 cup celery, diced
- 1/2 cup mayonnaise
- 1/8 tsp (dash) Tabasco sauce
- 2 lemon juice
- 1/4 tsp black pepper

Directions:

1. Combine the cooked chicken, pineapple, lettuce, and celery in a medium bowl. Just set aside.

2. In a small bowl, make the dressing. Mix the mayonnaise, Tabasco sauce, pepper, and lemon juice.

3. Use the chicken mixture to add the dressing and stir until well mixed.

Nutrition: Power: 310 g, Protein: 16.8 g, Carbohydrates: 9.6 g, fibbers: 1.1 g, Fat: 23.1 g, Sodium: 200 mg, Potassium: 260 mg, Phosphorus: 134 mg

FISH & SEAFOOD

Sardine Fish Cakes

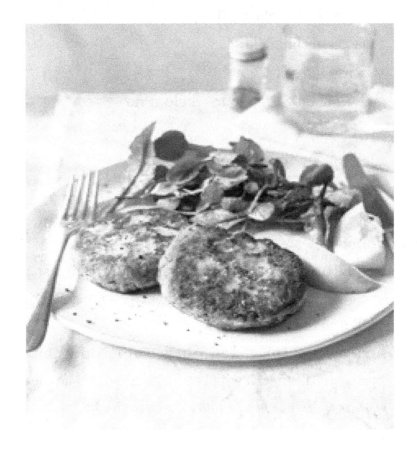

Preparation Time: 10 minutes

Cooking Time: 10 minutes

Servings: 4

Ingredients:

- 11 oz. sardines, canned, drained
- 1/3 cup shallot, chopped
- 1 teaspoon chili flakes
- ½ teaspoon salt
- 2 tablespoon wheat flour, whole grain
- 1 egg, beaten
- 1 tablespoon chives, chopped
- 1 teaspoon olive oil
- 1 teaspoon butter

Directions:

1. Put the butter in your skillet and dissolve it. Add shallot and cook it until translucent. After this, transfer the shallot to the mixing bowl.

2. Add sardines, chili flakes, salt, flour, egg, chives, and mix up until smooth with the fork's help. Make the medium size cakes and place them in the skillet. Add olive oil.

3. Roast the fish cakes for 3 minutes from each side over medium heat. Dry the cooked fish cakes with a paper towel if needed and transfer to the serving plates.

Nutrition: Calories 221Fat 12.2gFiber 0.1gCarbs 5.4g Protein 21.3 g Phosphorus 188.7 mg Potassium 160.3 mg Sodium 452.6 mg

4-Ingredients Salmon Fillet

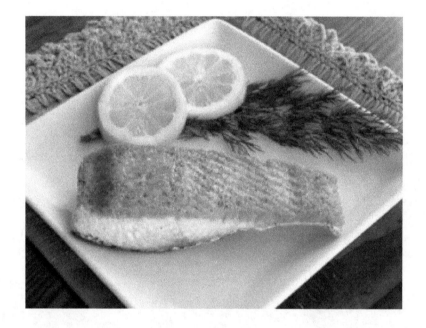

Preparation Time: 5 minutes

Cooking Time: 25 minutes

Servings: 1

Ingredients:

- 4 oz. salmon fillet
- ½ teaspoon salt
- 1 teaspoon sesame oil
- ½ teaspoon sage

Directions:

1. Rub the fillet with salt and sage. Put the fish in the tray, then sprinkle it with sesame oil. Cook the fish for 25 minutes at 365F. Flip the fish carefully onto another side after 12 minutes of cooking. Serve.

Nutrition: Calories 191Fat 11.6gFiber 0.1gCarbs 0.2gProtein 22g Sodium 70.5 mg Phosphorus 472 mg   Potassium 636.3 mg

Spanish Cod in Sauce

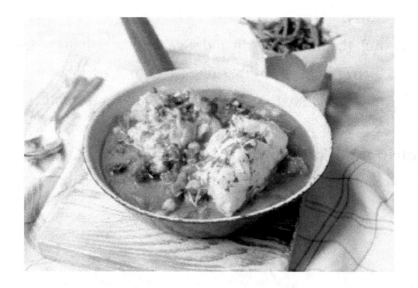

Preparation Time: 10 minutes

Cooking Time: 5 1/2 hours

Servings: 2

Ingredients:

- 1 teaspoon tomato paste
- 1 teaspoon garlic, diced
- 1 white onion, sliced
- 1 jalapeno pepper, chopped
- 1/3 cup chicken stock
- 7 oz. Spanish cod fillet
- 1 teaspoon paprika
- 1 teaspoon salt

Directions:

1. Pour chicken stock into the saucepan. Add tomato paste and mix up the liquid until homogenous. Add garlic, onion, jalapeno pepper, paprika, and salt.
2. Bring the liquid to boil and then simmer it. Chop the cod fillet and add it to the tomato liquid. Simmer the fish for 10 minutes over low heat. Serve the fish in the bowls with tomato sauce.

Nutrition: Calories 113 Fat 1.2g Fiber 1.9g Carbs 7.2g Protein 18.9g Potassium 659 mg Sodium 597 mg Phosphorus 18 mg

Salmon Baked in Foil with Fresh Thyme

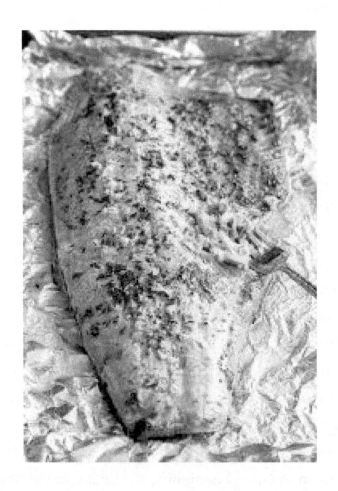

Preparation Time: 10 minutes

Cooking Time: 30 minutes

Servings: 4

Ingredients:

- 4 fresh thyme sprigs
- 4 garlic cloves, peeled, roughly chopped
- 16 oz. salmon fillets (4 oz. each fillet)
- ½ teaspoon salt
- ½ teaspoon ground black pepper
- 4 tablespoons cream
- 4 teaspoons butter
- ¼ teaspoon cumin seeds

Directions:

1. Line the baking tray with foil. Sprinkle the fish fillets with salt, ground black pepper, cumin seeds, and arrange them in the tray with oil.
2. Add thyme sprig on the top of every fillet. Then add cream, butter, and garlic. Bake the fish for 30 minutes at 345F. Serve.

Nutrition: Calories 198 Fat 11.6g Carbs 1.8g Protein 22.4g Phosphorus 425 mg Potassium 660.9 mg Sodium 366 mg

Poached Halibut in Mango Sauce

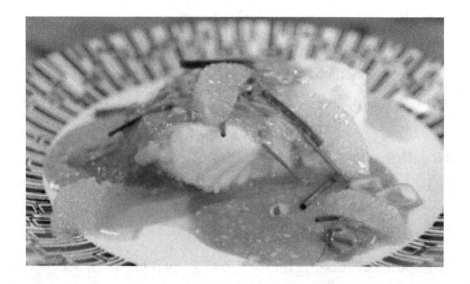

Preparation Time: 10 minutes

Cooking Time: 10 minutes

Servings: 4

Ingredients:

- 1-pound halibut
- 1/3 cup butter
- 1 rosemary sprig
- ½ teaspoon ground black pepper
- 1 teaspoon salt
- 1 teaspoon honey
- ¼ cup of mango juice
- 1 teaspoon cornstarch

Directions:

1. Put butter in the saucepan and melt it. Add rosemary sprig. Sprinkle the halibut with salt and ground black pepper. Put the fish in the boiling butter and poach it for 4 minutes.

2. Meanwhile, pour mango juice into the skillet. Add honey and bring the liquid to boil. Add cornstarch and whisk until the liquid starts to be thick. Then remove it from the heat.

3. Transfer the poached halibut to the plate and cut it on 4. Place every fish serving in the serving plate and top with mango sauce.

Nutrition: Calories 349 Fat 29.3g Fiber 0.1g Carbs 3.2g Protein 17.8g Phosphorus 154 mg Potassium 388.6 mg Sodium 29.3 mg

POULTRY RECIPES

Zucchini and turkey burger with jalapeno peppers

Preparation Time: 15 minutes

Cooking Time: 10 minutes

Servings: 4

Ingredients

- Turkey meat (ground) – 1 pound
- Zucchini (shredded) – 1 cup
- Onion (minced) – ½ cup
- Jalapeño pepper (seeded and minced) – 1
- Egg – 1
- Extra-spicy blend – 1 teaspoon
- Fresh polao peppers (seeded and sliced in half lengthwise)
- Mustard – 1 teaspoon

Directions

1. Start by taking a mixing bowl and adding in the turkey meat, zucchini, onion, jalapeño pepper, egg, and extra-spicy blend. Mix well to combine.

2. Divide the mixture into 4 equal portions. Form burger patties out of the same.

3. Prepare an electric griddle or an outdoor grill. Place the burger patties on the grill and cook until the top is blistered and tender. Place the sliced poblano peppers on the grill alongside the patties. Grilling the patties should take about 5 minutes on each side.

4. Once done, place the patties onto the buns and top them with grilled peppers.

Nutrition: protein – 25 g carbohydrates – 5 g fat – 10 g cholesterol – 125 mg sodium – 128 mg potassium – 475 mg phosphorus – 280 mg calcium – 43 mg fiber – 1.6 g name

Gnocchi and chicken dumplings

Preparation Time: 10 minutes

Cooking Time: 40 minutes

Servings: 10

Ingredients

- Chicken breast – 2 pounds
- Gnocchi – 1 pound
- Light olive oil – ¼ cup
- Better than bouillon® chicken base – 1 tablespoon
- Chicken stock (reduced-sodium) – 6 cups
- Fresh celery (diced finely) – ½ cup
- Fresh onions (diced finely) – ½ cup
- Fresh carrots (diced finely) – ½ cup
- Fresh parsley (chopped) – ¼ cup
- Black pepper – 1 teaspoon
- Italian seasoning – 1 teaspoon

Directions

1. Start by placing the stock over a high flame. Add in the oil and let it heat through.

2. Add the chicken to the hot oil and shallow-fry until all sides turn golden brown.

3. Toss in the carrots, onions, and celery and cook for about 5 minutes. Pour in the chicken stock and let it cool on a high flame for about 30 minutes.

4. Reduce the flame and add in the chicken bouillon, italian seasoning, and black pepper. Stir well.

5. Toss in the store-bought gnocchi and let it cook for about 15 minutes. Keep stirring.

6. Once done, transfer into a serving bowl. Add parsley and serve hot!

Nutrition: protein – 28 g carbohydrates – 38 g fat – 10 g cholesterol – 58 mg sodium – 121 mg potassium – 485 mg calcium – 38 mg fiber – 2 g

Creamy Turkey

Preparation Time: 12 minutes

Cooking Time: 10 minutes

Servings: 4

Ingredients:

- 4 skinless, boneless turkey breast halves
- Salt and pepper to taste
- ½ teaspoon ground black pepper
- ½ teaspoon garlic powder
- 1 (10.75 ounces) can chicken soup

Directions:

1. Preheat oven to 375 degrees F.

2. Clean turkey breasts and season with salt, pepper and garlic powder (or whichever seasonings you prefer) on both sides of turkey pieces.

3. Bake for 25 minutes, then add chicken soup and bake for 10 more minutes (or until done). Serve over rice or egg noodles.

Nutrition: Calories 160, Sodium 157mg, Dietary Fiber 0.4g, Total Sugars 0.4g, Protein 25.6g, Calcium 2mg, Potassium 152mg, Phosphorus 85 mg

MEAT RECIPES

Peppercorn Pork Chops

Preparation time: 30 min

Cooking Time: 30 minutes

Servings: 4

Ingredients:

- 1 tablespoon crushed black peppercorns
- 4 pork loin chops
- 2 tablespoons olive oil
- 1/4 cup butter
- 5 garlic cloves
- 1 cup green and red bell peppers
- 1/2 cup pineapple juice

Directions:

1. Sprinkle and press peppercorns into both sides of pork chops.

2. Heat oil, butter and garlic cloves in a large skillet over medium heat, stirring frequently.

3. Add pork chops and cook uncovered for 5–6 minutes.

4. Dice the bell peppers. Add the bell peppers and pineapple juice to the pork chops.

5. Cover and simmer for another 5–6 minutes or until pork is thoroughly cooked.

Nutrition: Calories 317, Total Fat 25.7g, Saturated Fat 10.5g, Cholesterol 66mg, Sodium 126mg, Total Carbohydrate 9.2g, Dietary Fiber 2g, Total Sugars 6.4g, Protein 13.2g, Calcium 39mg, Iron 1mg, Potassium 250mg, Phosphorus 115 mg

Pork Chops with Apples, Onions

Preparation time: 30 min

Cooking Time: 60 minutes

Servings: 4

Ingredients:

- 4 pork chops
- salt and pepper to taste
- 2 onions, sliced into rings
- 2 apples - peeled, cored, and sliced into rings
- 3 tablespoons honey
- 2 teaspoons freshly ground black pepper

Directions:

1. Preheat oven to 375 degrees F.

2. Season pork chops with salt and pepper to taste, and arrange in a medium oven-safe skillet. Top pork chops with onions and apples. Sprinkle with honey. Season with 2 teaspoons pepper.

3. Cover, and bake 1 hour in the preheated oven, pork chops have reached an internal temperature of 145 degrees F.

Nutrition: Calories 307, Total Fat 16.1g, Saturated Fat 6g, Cholesterol 55mg, Sodium 48mg, Total Carbohydrate 26.8g, Dietary Fiber 3.1g, Total Sugars 21.5g, Protein 15.1g, Calcium 30mg, Iron 1mg, Potassium 387mg, Phosphorus 315 mg

BROTHS, CONDIMENT AND SEASONING

Spicy Herb Seasoning

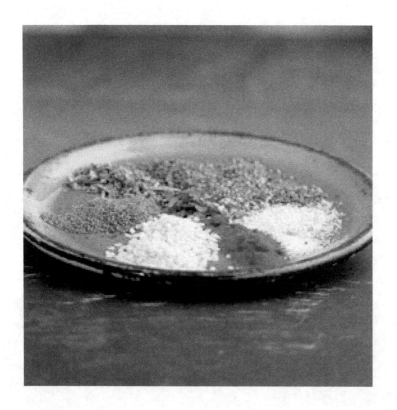

Preparation Time: 10 minutes

Cooking Time: 0 minutes

Servings: ½ cup

Ingredients:

- ¼ cup celery seed
- 1 tablespoon dried basil
- 1 tablespoon dried oregano
- 1 tablespoon dried thyme
- 1 tablespoon onion powder
- 2 teaspoons garlic powder
- 1 teaspoon freshly ground black pepper
- ½ teaspoon ground cloves

Directions:

1. Mix the celery seed, basil, oregano, thyme, onion powder, garlic powder, pepper, and cloves in a small bowl. Store for up to 1 month.

Nutrition: Calories: 7 Fat: 0g Sodium: 2mg Carbohydrates: 1g

Phosphorus: 9mg Potassium: 27mg Protein: 0g

Phosphorus-Free Baking Powder

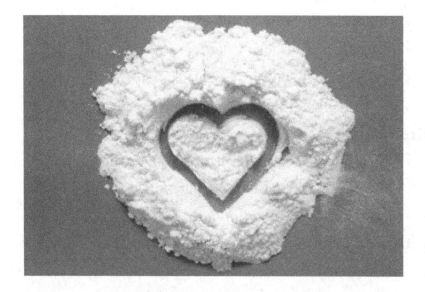

Preparation Time: 5 minutes

Cooking Time: 0 minutes

Servings: 1

Ingredients:

- ¾ cup cream of tartar
- ¼ cup baking soda

Directions:

1. Mix the cream of tartar plus baking soda in a small bowl. Sift the mixture together several times to mix thoroughly. Store the baking powder in a sealed container in a cool, dark place for up to 1 month.

Nutrition: Calories: 6 Fat: 0g Sodium: 309mg Carbohydrates: 1g Phosphorus: 0g Potassium: 341mg Protein: 0g

DRINKS AND SMOOTHIES

Almonds & Blueberries Smoothie

Preparation Time: 5 minutes

Cooking Time: 3 minutes

Servings: 2

Ingredients:

- 1/4 cup ground almonds, unsalted
- 1 cup fresh blueberries
- Fresh juice of a 1 lemon
- 1 cup fresh kale leaf
- 1/2 cup coconut water
- 1 cup water
- 2 tablespoon plain yogurt (optional)

Directions:

1. Dump all ingredients in your high-speed blender, and blend until your smoothie is smooth.

2. Pour the mixture in a chilled glass.

3. Serve and enjoy!

Nutrition: Calories: 110, Carbohydrates: 8g, Proteins: 2g, Fat: 7g, Fiber: 2g, Calcium 19mg, Phosphorous 16mg, Potassium 27mg Sodium: 101 mg

Almonds and Zucchini Smoothie

Preparation Time: 5 minutes

Cooking Time: 3 minutes

Servings: 2

Ingredients:

- 1 cup zucchini, cooked and mashed - unsalted
- 1 1/2 cups almond milk
- 1 tablespoon almond butter (plain, unsalted)
- 1 teaspoon pure almond extract
- 2 tablespoon ground almonds or macadamia almonds
- 1/2 cup water
- 1 cup ice cubes crushed (optional, for serving)

Directions:

1. Dump all ingredients from the list above in your fast-speed blender; blend for 45 - 60 seconds or to taste.

2. Serve with crushed ice.

Nutrition: Calories: 322, Carbohydrates: 6g, Proteins: 6g, Fat: 30g, Fiber: 3.5g Calcium 9mg, Phosphorous 26mg, Potassium 27mg Sodium: 121 mg

DESSERT

Baked apples with cherries and walnuts

Preparation time: 10 minutes

Cooking time: 35 to 40 minutes

Servings: 6

Ingredients:

- 1/3 cup dried cherries, coarsely chopped
- 3 tablespoons chopped walnuts
- 1 tablespoon ground flaxseed meal
- 1 tablespoon firmly packed brown sugar
- 1 teaspoon ground cinnamon
- 1/8 teaspoon nutmeg
- 6 golden delicious apples, about 2 pounds total weight, washed and unpeeled
- 1/2 cup 100 percent apple juice
- 1/4 cup water
- 2 tablespoons dark honey
- 2 teaspoons extra-virgin olive oil

Directions:

1. Preheat the oven to 350°f.

2. In a small bowl, toss together the cherries, walnuts, flaxseed meal, brown sugar, cinnamon, and nutmeg until all the ingredients are evenly distributed. Set aside.

3. Working from the stem end, core each apple, stopping ¾ of an inch from the bottom.

4. Gently press the cherries into each apple cavity. Arrange the apples upright in a heavy ovenproof skillet or baking dish just large enough to hold them.

5. Pour the apple juice and water into the pan.

6. Drizzle the honey and oil evenly over the apples, and cover the pan snugly with aluminum foil. Bake until the apples are tender when pierced with a knife, 35 to 40 minutes.

7. Transfer the apples to individual plates and drizzle with the pan juices. Serve warm.

Nutrition: calories: 162; total fat 5g; saturated fat: 1g; cholesterol: 0mg; sodium: 4mg; potassium: 148mg; total carbohydrate: 30g; fiber: 4g; protein: 1g

Easy peach crumble

Preparation time: 10 minutes

Cooking time: 30 minutes

Servings: 8

Ingredients:

- 8 ripe peaches, peeled, pitted and sliced
- 3 tablespoons freshly squeezed lemon juice
- 1/2 teaspoon ground cinnamon
- 1/4 teaspoon ground nutmeg
- 1/2 cup oat flour
- 1/4 cup packed dark brown sugar
- 2 tablespoons margarine, cut into thin slices
- 1/4 cup quick-cooking oats

Directions:

1. Preheat the oven to 375°f. Lightly coat a 9-inch pie pan with cooking spray. Arrange peach slices in the prepared pie plate and sprinkle with the lemon juice, cinnamon, and nutmeg.

2. In a small bowl, whisk together the flour and brown sugar. With your fingers, crumble the margarine into the flour-sugar mixture. Add the uncooked oats and stir to mix. Sprinkle the flour mixture over the peaches.

3. Bake until the peaches are soft and the topping is browned, about 30 minutes.

4. Cut into 8 even slices and serve warm.

Nutrition: calories: 130; total fat 4g; saturated fat: 0g; cholesterol: 0mg; sodium: 42mg; potassium: 255mg; total carbohydrate: 28g; fiber: 3g; protein: 2g

Lemon thins

Preparation time: 15 minutes

Cooking time: 8 to 10 minutes

Servings: 30 cookies

Ingredients:

- Cooking spray
- 11/4 cups whole wheat pastry flour
- 1/3 cup cornstarch
- 11/2 teaspoons baking powder
- ¾ cup sugar, divided
- 2 tablespoons butter, softened
- 2 tablespoons extra-virgin olive oil
- 1 large egg white
- 3 teaspoons freshly grated lemon zest
- 11/2 teaspoons vanilla extract
- 4 tablespoons freshly squeezed lemon juice

Directions:

1. Preheat the oven to 350°f. Coat two baking sheets with cooking spray.

2. In a mixing bowl, whisk together the flour, cornstarch, and baking powder.

3. In another mixing bowl beat 1/2 cup of the sugar, the butter, and olive oil with an electric mixer on medium speed until fluffy.

4. Add the egg white, lemon zest, and vanilla and beat until smooth. Beat in the lemon juice.

5. Add the dry ingredients to the wet ingredients and fold in with a rubber spatula just until combined.

6. Drop the dough by the teaspoonful, 2 inches apart, onto the prepared baking sheets.

7. Place the remaining 1/4 cup sugar in a saucer. Coat the bottom of a wide-bottomed glass with cooking spray and dip it in the sugar. Flatten the dough with the glass bottom into 21/2-inch circles, dipping the glass in the sugar each time.

8. Bake the cookies until they are just starting to brown around the edges, 8 to 10 minutes. Transfer to a flat surface (not a rack) to crisp.

Nutrition: (1 cookie) calories: 40; total fat 2g; saturated fat: 1g; cholesterol: 2mg; sodium: 26mg; potassium: 3mg; total carbohydrate: 5g; fiber: 1g; protein: 1g